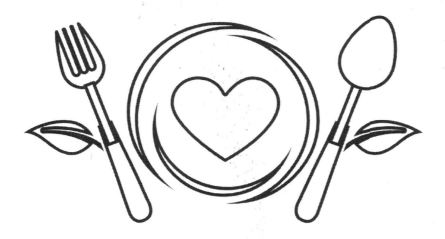

This Book Belongs To

_____

Stages of Hunger

1 - Not hungry at all
2 - A little hungry
3 - Hungry
4 - Painfully hungry

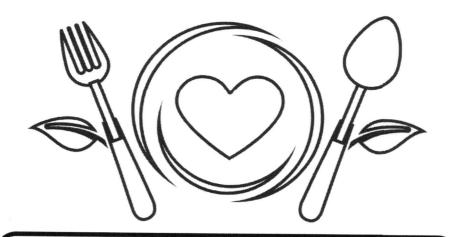

Stages of Fullness

1 - Not at all full
2 - Satisfied
3 - Full
4 - Painfully full

12 / 12 / 19

Food	Time	Hunger Level	Fullness Level	Emotion Before Eating	Emotion After Eating
donut	7:30	1	1	stressed	guilt
salad	11:45	3	2	none	pride
cheetos	1:15	1	4	bored sleepy	guilt
oreos	1:15	1	4	bored sleepy	guilt
chicken rice casserole	6:00	1	4	none	guilt

EXAMPLE

Drink (non-water)

	Time	Hunger Level	Fullness Level	Emotion Before Eating	Emotion After Eating
starbucks grande mocha latte	7:30	1	1	stressed	guilt
20 oz soda	1:15	1	4	bored sleepy	guilt

Exercise- (YES) NO   Water ___80___ OZ

Exercise Type___HIIT___   Wake Time ___6:15 am___

How Long?___12 min___   Bed Time ___11:15 pm___

How do I feel about today?
I woke up late today and didn't get a chance to make a healthy breakfast. Then I got bored and sleepy at work so I mindlessly snacked just to stay awake. Dinner was homemade, which made me feel good, but then I finished my second helping which made me feel overly full. But I did a workout today so I was pretty proud of myself for that. I'll use my affirmations to help me through my bored eating tomorrow.

What does Natural Hunger feel like to me?

Take a moment to write down what a non-emotional hunger feels like to help you recognize it when it shows up in your life.

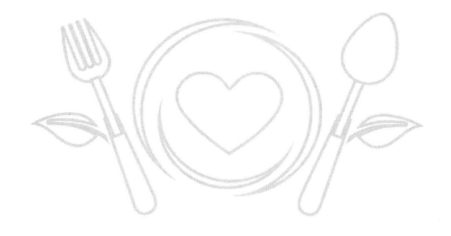

Affirmations to help with Emotional Eating

Here are some affirmations to help you get started on your journey. Make sure to write down new ones that you may come across that make you feel better about yourself.

I eat slowly and stop eating the moment I feel full.

I give myself permission to eat in a way that is good for my body and my mind.

I have the power to eat slowly and thoughtfully.

10 / 12 / 2020

Food	Time	Hunger Level	Fullness Level	Emotion Before Eating	Emotion After Eating
pb ~~beach~~ beachbar	6:00	3	3	okay	satisfied
McDonalds	12:00	3	4	relieved- good session	not as guilty as supposed to feel for eating th
misc snacks	4:00+	2	4		meh
dinner - chic salad	6:00	4	4		

Drink (non-water)

Drink	Time	Hunger Level	Fullness Level	Emotion Before Eating	Emotion After Eating
Coffee w/ 1 sugar + pumpkin creamer	6:00	3	3	sleepy/ okay/	good-not too antsy

Exercise- (YES) NO   Water _____ oz

Exercise Type 21DF   Wake Time 4:45

How Long? 30 min   Bed Time _____

How do I feel about today?

__ / __ / __

Food	Time	Hunger Level	Fullness Level	Emotion Before Eating	Emotion After Eating

Drink (non-water)

Exercise- YES   NO

Exercise Type_____

How Long?_____

Water _____oz

Wake Time _____

Bed Time _____

How do I feel about today?

___/___/___

Food	Time	Hunger Level	Fullness Level	Emotion Before Eating	Emotion After Eating

Drink (non-water)

Exercise- YES   NO   Water _____oz

Exercise Type_____   Wake Time _____

How Long?_____   Bed Time _____

How do I feel about today?

__/__/__

Food	Time	Hunger Level	Fullness Level	Emotion Before Eating	Emotion After Eating

Drink (non-water)

Exercise- YES   NO

Exercise Type_____

How Long?_____

Water _____oz

Wake Time _____

Bed Time _____

How do I feel about today?

__/__/__ Food	Time	Hunger Level	Fullness Level	Emotion Before Eating	Emotion After Eating

Drink (non-water)

Exercise- YES   NO   Water _____oz

Exercise Type_____   Wake Time _____

How Long?_____   Bed Time _____

How do I feel about today?

___ / ___ / ___

Food	Time	Hunger Level	Fullness Level	Emotion Before Eating	Emotion After Eating

Drink (non-water)

Exercise- YES   NO

Exercise Type_____

How Long?_____

Water _____oz

Wake Time _____

Bed Time _____

How do I feel about today?

___ / ___ / ___

Food	Time	Hunger Level	Fullness Level	Emotion Before Eating	Emotion After Eating

Drink (non-water)

	Time	Hunger Level	Fullness Level	Emotion Before Eating	Emotion After Eating

Exercise- YES   NO   Water _____ oz

Exercise Type_____   Wake Time _____

How Long?_____   Bed Time _____

How do I feel about today?

__/__/__

Food	Time	Hunger Level	Fullness Level	Emotion Before Eating	Emotion After Eating

Drink (non-water)

	Time	Hunger Level	Fullness Level	Emotion Before Eating	Emotion After Eating

Exercise- YES   NO

Exercise Type_____

How Long?_____

Water _____oz

Wake Time _____

Bed Time _____

How do I feel about today?

__/__/__ Food	Time	Hunger Level	Fullness Level	Emotion Before Eating	Emotion After Eating

Drink (non-water)

Exercise- YES   NO

Exercise Type_____

How Long?_____

Water _____oz

Wake Time _____

Bed Time _____

How do I feel about today?

_ _ / _ _ / _ _

Food	Time	Hunger Level	Fullness Level	Emotion Before Eating	Emotion After Eating

Drink (non-water)

Exercise- YES   NO

Exercise Type_____

How Long?_____

Water _____oz

Wake Time _____

Bed Time _____

How do I feel about today?

___ / ___ / ___

Food		Time	Hunger Level	Fullness Level	Emotion Before Eating	Emotion After Eating

Drink (non-water)

Exercise- YES   NO   Water _____ oz

Exercise Type_____   Wake Time _____

How Long?_____   Bed Time _____

How do I feel about today?

___/___/___

Food	Time	Hunger Level	Fullness Level	Emotion Before Eating	Emotion After Eating

Drink (non-water)

Exercise- YES   NO   Water _____oz

Exercise Type_____   Wake Time _____

How Long?_____   Bed Time _____

How do I feel about today?

___/___/___

Food	Time	Hunger Level	Fullness Level	Emotion Before Eating	Emotion After Eating

Drink (non-water)

Exercise- YES   NO

Exercise Type_____

How Long?_____

Water _____oz

Wake Time _____

Bed Time _____

How do I feel about today?

___/___/___

Food	Time	Hunger Level	Fullness Level	Emotion Before Eating	Emotion After Eating

Drink (non-water)

Exercise- YES   NO

Exercise Type_____

How Long?_____

Water _____oz

Wake Time _____

Bed Time _____

How do I feel about today?

___/___/___

Food	Time	Hunger Level	Fullness Level	Emotion Before Eating	Emotion After Eating

Drink (non-water)

Exercise- YES   NO

Exercise Type_____

How Long?_____

Water _____oz

Wake Time _____

Bed Time _____

How do I feel about today?

___/___/___

Food	Time	Hunger Level	Fullness Level	Emotion Before Eating	Emotion After Eating

Drink (non-water)

Exercise- YES   NO

Exercise Type_____

How Long?_____

Water _____oz

Wake Time _____

Bed Time _____

How do I feel about today?

___/___/___

Food	Time	Hunger Level	Fullness Level	Emotion Before Eating	Emotion After Eating

Drink (non-water)

Exercise- YES   NO   Water _____oz

Exercise Type_____   Wake Time _____

How Long?_____   Bed Time _____

How do I feel about today?

___/___/___

Food	Time	Hunger Level	Fullness Level	Emotion Before Eating	Emotion After Eating

Drink (non-water)

Exercise- YES   NO

Exercise Type_____

How Long?_____

Water _____oz

Wake Time _____

Bed Time _____

How do I feel about today?

___/___/___

Food	Time	Hunger Level	Fullness Level	Emotion Before Eating	Emotion After Eating

Drink (non-water)

Exercise- YES   NO   Water _____oz
Exercise Type_____   Wake Time _____
How Long?_____   Bed Time _____

How do I feel about today?

__ / __ / __

Food	Time	Hunger Level	Fullness Level	Emotion Before Eating	Emotion After Eating

Drink (non-water)

Exercise- YES   NO

Exercise Type_____

How Long?_____

Water _____ oz

Wake Time _____

Bed Time _____

How do I feel about today?

___/___/___

Food	Time	Hunger Level	Fullness Level	Emotion Before Eating	Emotion After Eating

Drink (non-water)

Exercise- YES   NO
Exercise Type_____
How Long?_____

Water _____oz
Wake Time _____
Bed Time _____

How do I feel about today?

___ / ___ / ___

Food	Time	Hunger Level	Fullness Level	Emotion Before Eating	Emotion After Eating

Drink (non-water)					

Exercise- YES   NO

Exercise Type_____

How Long?_____

Water _____oz

Wake Time _____

Bed Time _____

How do I feel about today?

___/___/___

Food	Time	Hunger Level	Fullness Level	Emotion Before Eating	Emotion After Eating

Drink (non-water)

Exercise- YES   NO   Water _____oz
Exercise Type_____   Wake Time _____
How Long?_____   Bed Time _____

How do I feel about today?

___/___/___

Food	Time	Hunger Level	Fullness Level	Emotion Before Eating	Emotion After Eating

Drink (non-water)

Exercise- YES   NO

Exercise Type_____

How Long?_____

Water _____oz

Wake Time _____

Bed Time _____

How do I feel about today?

___/___/___

Food	Time	Hunger Level	Fullness Level	Emotion Before Eating	Emotion After Eating

Drink (non-water)

	Time	Hunger Level	Fullness Level	Emotion Before Eating	Emotion After Eating

Exercise- YES   NO   Water _____oz

Exercise Type_____   Wake Time _____

How Long?_____   Bed Time _____

How do I feel about today?

___/___/___

Food	Time	Hunger Level	Fullness Level	Emotion Before Eating	Emotion After Eating

Drink (non-water)

	Time	Hunger Level	Fullness Level	Emotion Before Eating	Emotion After Eating

Exercise- YES   NO

Exercise Type_____

How Long?_____

Water _____oz

Wake Time _____

Bed Time _____

How do I feel about today?

___/___/___

Food	Time	Hunger Level	Fullness Level	Emotion Before Eating	Emotion After Eating

Drink (non-water)

Exercise- YES   NO   Water _____oz
Exercise Type_____   Wake Time _____
How Long?_____   Bed Time _____

How do I feel about today?

___ / ___ / ___

Food		Time	Hunger Level	Fullness Level	Emotion Before Eating	Emotion After Eating

Drink (non-water)

Exercise- YES   NO

Exercise Type_____

How Long?_____

Water _____oz

Wake Time _____

Bed Time _____

How do I feel about today?

___/___/___

Food	Time	Hunger Level	Fullness Level	Emotion Before Eating	Emotion After Eating

Drink (non-water)

Exercise- YES   NO

Exercise Type_____

How Long?_____

Water _____oz

Wake Time _____

Bed Time _____

How do I feel about today?

___ / ___ / ___

Food	Time	Hunger Level	Fullness Level	Emotion Before Eating	Emotion After Eating

Drink (non-water)

Exercise- YES   NO

Exercise Type_____

How Long?_____

Water _____ oz

Wake Time _____

Bed Time _____

How do I feel about today?

___ / ___ / ___

Food	Time	Hunger Level	Fullness Level	Emotion Before Eating	Emotion After Eating

Drink (non-water)

Exercise- YES   NO   Water _____oz

Exercise Type_____   Wake Time _____

How Long?_____   Bed Time _____

How do I feel about today?

___/___/___

Food	Time	Hunger Level	Fullness Level	Emotion Before Eating	Emotion After Eating

Drink (non-water)

Exercise- YES   NO

Exercise Type_____

How Long?_____

Water _____oz

Wake Time _____

Bed Time _____

How do I feel about today?

__/__/__ Food	Time	Hunger Level	Fullness Level	Emotion Before Eating	Emotion After Eating

Drink (non-water)

Exercise- YES NO   Water _____oz
Exercise Type_____   Wake Time _____
How Long?_____   Bed Time _____

How do I feel about today?

__ / __ / __

Food	Time	Hunger Level	Fullness Level	Emotion Before Eating	Emotion After Eating

Drink (non-water)					

Exercise- YES   NO

Exercise Type_____

How Long?_____

Water _____oz

Wake Time _____

Bed Time _____

How do I feel about today?

__ / __ / __

Food	Time	Hunger Level	Fullness Level	Emotion Before Eating	Emotion After Eating

Drink (non-water)

Exercise- YES   NO   Water _____oz

Exercise Type_____   Wake Time _____

How Long?_____   Bed Time _____

How do I feel about today?

__/__/__

Food	Time	Hunger Level	Fullness Level	Emotion Before Eating	Emotion After Eating

Drink (non-water)

Exercise- YES   NO

Exercise Type_____

How Long?_____

Water _____oz

Wake Time _____

Bed Time _____

How do I feel about today?

___ / ___ / ___

Food	Time	Hunger Level	Fullness Level	Emotion Before Eating	Emotion After Eating

Drink (non-water)

Exercise- YES   NO

Exercise Type_____

How Long?_____

Water _____oz

Wake Time _____

Bed Time _____

How do I feel about today?

__/__/__

Food	Time	Hunger Level	Fullness Level	Emotion Before Eating	Emotion After Eating

Drink (non-water)					

Exercise- YES   NO

Exercise Type_____

How Long?_____

Water _____oz

Wake Time _____

Bed Time _____

How do I feel about today?

___/___/___

Food	Time	Hunger Level	Fullness Level	Emotion Before Eating	Emotion After Eating

Drink (non-water)

Exercise- YES   NO   Water _____oz

Exercise Type_____   Wake Time _____

How Long?_____   Bed Time _____

How do I feel about today?

__/__/__ Food	Time	Hunger Level	Fullness Level	Emotion Before Eating	Emotion After Eating

Drink (non-water)

Exercise- YES   NO

Exercise Type_____

How Long?_____

Water _____oz

Wake Time _____

Bed Time _____

How do I feel about today?

___/___/___

Food

	Time	Hunger Level	Fullness Level	Emotion Before Eating	Emotion After Eating

Drink (non-water)

Exercise- YES   NO   Water _____oz

Exercise Type_____   Wake Time _____

How Long?_____   Bed Time _____

How do I feel about today?

__/__/__ Food	Time	Hunger Level	Fullness Level	Emotion Before Eating	Emotion After Eating

Drink (non-water)

Exercise- YES   NO   Water _____oz

Exercise Type_____   Wake Time _____

How Long?_____   Bed Time _____

How do I feel about today?

___/___/___

Food	Time	Hunger Level	Fullness Level	Emotion Before Eating	Emotion After Eating

Drink (non-water)

	Time	Hunger Level	Fullness Level	Emotion Before Eating	Emotion After Eating

Exercise- YES   NO

Exercise Type_____

How Long?_____

Water _____oz

Wake Time _____

Bed Time _____

How do I feel about today?

___ / ___ / ___

Food	Time	Hunger Level	Fullness Level	Emotion Before Eating	Emotion After Eating

Drink (non-water)

Exercise- YES   NO

Exercise Type_____

How Long?_____

Water _____oz

Wake Time _____

Bed Time _____

How do I feel about today?

___/___/___

Food	Time	Hunger Level	Fullness Level	Emotion Before Eating	Emotion After Eating

Drink (non-water)

Exercise- YES   NO

Exercise Type_____

How Long?_____

Water _____oz

Wake Time _____

Bed Time _____

How do I feel about today?

___/___/___

Food	Time	Hunger Level	Fullness Level	Emotion Before Eating	Emotion After Eating

Drink (non-water)

Exercise- YES   NO

Exercise Type_____

How Long?_____

Water _____oz

Wake Time _____

Bed Time _____

How do I feel about today?

__ / __ / __

Food	Time	Hunger Level	Fullness Level	Emotion Before Eating	Emotion After Eating

Drink (non-water)

Exercise- YES   NO

Exercise Type_____

How Long?_____

Water _____oz

Wake Time _____

Bed Time _____

How do I feel about today?

___/___/___

Food	Time	Hunger Level	Fullness Level	Emotion Before Eating	Emotion After Eating

Drink (non-water)

Exercise- YES   NO

Exercise Type_____

How Long?_____

Water _____oz

Wake Time _____

Bed Time _____

How do I feel about today?

__/__/__ Food	Time	Hunger Level	Fullness Level	Emotion Before Eating	Emotion After Eating

Drink (non-water)

Exercise- YES   NO

Exercise Type_____

How Long?_____

Water _____oz

Wake Time _____

Bed Time _____

How do I feel about today?

__/__/__ Food	Time	Hunger Level	Fullness Level	Emotion Before Eating	Emotion After Eating

Drink (non-water)

Exercise- YES   NO

Exercise Type_____

How Long?_____

Water _____oz

Wake Time _____

Bed Time _____

How do I feel about today?

__ / __ / __

Food	Time	Hunger Level	Fullness Level	Emotion Before Eating	Emotion After Eating

Drink (non-water)

Exercise- YES   NO   Water _____oz
Exercise Type_____   Wake Time _____
How Long?_____   Bed Time _____

How do I feel about today?

__ / __ / __

Food	Time	Hunger Level	Fullness Level	Emotion Before Eating	Emotion After Eating

Drink (non-water)

	Time	Hunger Level	Fullness Level	Emotion Before Eating	Emotion After Eating

Exercise- YES   NO

Exercise Type_____

How Long?_____

Water _____oz

Wake Time _____

Bed Time _____

How do I feel about today?

___ / ___ / ___

Food	Time	Hunger Level	Fullness Level	Emotion Before Eating	Emotion After Eating

Drink (non-water)

Exercise- YES   NO   Water _____oz

Exercise Type_____   Wake Time _____

How Long?_____   Bed Time _____

How do I feel about today?

___/___/___

Food	Time	Hunger Level	Fullness Level	Emotion Before Eating	Emotion After Eating

Drink (non-water)

Exercise- YES   NO

Exercise Type_____

How Long?_____

Water _____oz

Wake Time _____

Bed Time _____

How do I feel about today?

__ / __ / __

Food	Time	Hunger Level	Fullness Level	Emotion Before Eating	Emotion After Eating

Drink (non-water)

Exercise- YES   NO

Exercise Type_____

How Long?_____

Water _____oz

Wake Time _____

Bed Time _____

How do I feel about today?

___/___/___

Food	Time	Hunger Level	Fullness Level	Emotion Before Eating	Emotion After Eating

Drink (non-water)

	Time	Hunger Level	Fullness Level	Emotion Before Eating	Emotion After Eating

Exercise- YES   NO

Exercise Type_____

How Long?_____

Water _____oz

Wake Time _____

Bed Time _____

How do I feel about today?

___/___/___

Food	Time	Hunger Level	Fullness Level	Emotion Before Eating	Emotion After Eating

Drink (non-water)

Exercise- YES   NO   Water _____oz
Exercise Type_____   Wake Time _____
How Long?_____   Bed Time _____

How do I feel about today?

__ / __ / __

Food	Time	Hunger Level	Fullness Level	Emotion Before Eating	Emotion After Eating

Drink (non-water)

Exercise- YES   NO

Exercise Type_____

How Long?_____

Water _____oz

Wake Time _____

Bed Time _____

How do I feel about today?

___/___/___

Food	Time	Hunger Level	Fullness Level	Emotion Before Eating	Emotion After Eating

Drink (non-water)

	Time	Hunger Level	Fullness Level	Emotion Before Eating	Emotion After Eating

Exercise- YES   NO   Water _____oz

Exercise Type_____   Wake Time _____

How Long?_____   Bed Time _____

How do I feel about today?

___/___/___

Food	Time	Hunger Level	Fullness Level	Emotion Before Eating	Emotion After Eating

Drink (non-water)

	Time	Hunger Level	Fullness Level	Emotion Before Eating	Emotion After Eating

Exercise- YES   NO

Exercise Type_____

How Long?_____

Water _____oz

Wake Time _____

Bed Time _____

How do I feel about today?

___/___/___

Food	Time	Hunger Level	Fullness Level	Emotion Before Eating	Emotion After Eating

Drink (non-water)

Exercise- YES   NO   Water _____oz

Exercise Type_____   Wake Time _____

How Long?_____   Bed Time _____

How do I feel about today?

___/___/___

Food	Time	Hunger Level	Fullness Level	Emotion Before Eating	Emotion After Eating

Drink (non-water)

Exercise- YES   NO

Exercise Type_____

How Long?_____

Water _____oz

Wake Time _____

Bed Time _____

How do I feel about today?

___/___/___

Food	Time	Hunger Level	Fullness Level	Emotion Before Eating	Emotion After Eating

Drink (non-water)

Exercise- YES   NO

Exercise Type_____

How Long?_____

Water _____oz

Wake Time _____

Bed Time _____

How do I feel about today?

___/___/___

Food	Time	Hunger Level	Fullness Level	Emotion Before Eating	Emotion After Eating

Drink (non-water)

Exercise- YES   NO

Exercise Type_____

How Long?_____

Water _____oz

Wake Time _____

Bed Time _____

How do I feel about today?

___/___/___

Food

	Time	Hunger Level	Fullness Level	Emotion Before Eating	Emotion After Eating

Drink (non-water)

Exercise- YES   NO   Water _____oz
Exercise Type_____   Wake Time _____
How Long?_____   Bed Time _____

How do I feel about today?

__ / __ / __

Food	Time	Hunger Level	Fullness Level	Emotion Before Eating	Emotion After Eating

Drink (non-water)

Exercise- YES   NO

Exercise Type_____

How Long?_____

Water _____oz

Wake Time _____

Bed Time _____

How do I feel about today?

__/__/__ Food	Time	Hunger Level	Fullness Level	Emotion Before Eating	Emotion After Eating

Drink (non-water)

Exercise- YES   NO

Exercise Type_____

How Long?_____

Water _____oz

Wake Time _____

Bed Time _____

How do I feel about today?

___ / ___ / ___

Food	Time	Hunger Level	Fullness Level	Emotion Before Eating	Emotion After Eating

Drink (non-water)

Exercise- YES   NO

Exercise Type_____

How Long?_____

Water _____oz

Wake Time _____

Bed Time _____

How do I feel about today?

___/___/___

Food	Time	Hunger Level	Fullness Level	Emotion Before Eating	Emotion After Eating

Drink (non-water)

Exercise- YES   NO

Exercise Type_____

How Long?_____

Water _____oz

Wake Time _____

Bed Time _____

How do I feel about today?

___ / ___ / ___ Food	Time	Hunger Level	Fullness Level	Emotion Before Eating	Emotion After Eating

Drink (non-water)

Exercise- YES   NO   Water _____ oz

Exercise Type_____   Wake Time _____

How Long?_____   Bed Time _____

How do I feel about today?

___/___/___

Food	Time	Hunger Level	Fullness Level	Emotion Before Eating	Emotion After Eating

Drink (non-water)

Exercise- YES   NO

Exercise Type_____

How Long?_____

Water _____oz

Wake Time _____

Bed Time _____

How do I feel about today?

___ / ___ / ___

Food	Time	Hunger Level	Fullness Level	Emotion Before Eating	Emotion After Eating

Drink (non-water)

Exercise- YES   NO

Exercise Type_____

How Long?_____

Water _____oz

Wake Time _____

Bed Time _____

How do I feel about today?

___/___/___

Food	Time	Hunger Level	Fullness Level	Emotion Before Eating	Emotion After Eating

Drink (non-water)

Exercise- YES   NO

Exercise Type_____

How Long?_____

Water _____oz

Wake Time _____

Bed Time _____

How do I feel about today?

__/__/__

Food	Time	Hunger Level	Fullness Level	Emotion Before Eating	Emotion After Eating

Drink (non-water)

Exercise- YES   NO   Water _____ oz
Exercise Type_____   Wake Time _____
How Long?_____   Bed Time _____

How do I feel about today?

___/___/___

Food

	Time	Hunger Level	Fullness Level	Emotion Before Eating	Emotion After Eating

Drink (non-water)

Exercise- YES   NO

Exercise Type_____

How Long?_____

Water _____oz

Wake Time _____

Bed Time _____

How do I feel about today?

___/___/___

Food	Time	Hunger Level	Fullness Level	Emotion Before Eating	Emotion After Eating

Drink (non-water)

Exercise- YES   NO

Exercise Type_____

How Long?_____

Water _____oz

Wake Time _____

Bed Time _____

How do I feel about today?

___/___/___

Food	Time	Hunger Level	Fullness Level	Emotion Before Eating	Emotion After Eating

Drink (non-water)

Exercise- YES   NO

Exercise Type_____

How Long?_____

Water _____oz

Wake Time _____

Bed Time _____

How do I feel about today?

___ / ___ / ___

Food	Time	Hunger Level	Fullness Level	Emotion Before Eating	Emotion After Eating

Drink (non-water)

Exercise- YES   NO

Exercise Type_____

How Long?_____

Water _____oz

Wake Time _____

Bed Time _____

How do I feel about today?

___/___/___

Food	Time	Hunger Level	Fullness Level	Emotion Before Eating	Emotion After Eating

Drink (non-water)

Exercise- YES   NO

Exercise Type_____

How Long?_____

Water _____oz

Wake Time _____

Bed Time _____

How do I feel about today?

____/____/____

Food	Time	Hunger Level	Fullness Level	Emotion Before Eating	Emotion After Eating

Drink (non-water)

	Time	Hunger Level	Fullness Level	Emotion Before Eating	Emotion After Eating

Exercise- YES   NO   Water _____oz
Exercise Type_____   Wake Time _____
How Long?_____   Bed Time _____

How do I feel about today?

__/__/__

Food

	Time	Hunger Level	Fullness Level	Emotion Before Eating	Emotion After Eating

Drink (non-water)

Exercise- YES   NO

Exercise Type_____

How Long?_____

Water _____oz

Wake Time _____

Bed Time _____

How do I feel about today?

_ / _ / _

Food	Time	Hunger Level	Fullness Level	Emotion Before Eating	Emotion After Eating

Drink (non-water)

Exercise- YES   NO

Exercise Type_____

How Long?_____

Water _____oz

Wake Time _____

Bed Time _____

How do I feel about today?

__/__/__

Food	Time	Hunger Level	Fullness Level	Emotion Before Eating	Emotion After Eating

Drink (non-water)

Exercise- YES   NO

Exercise Type_____

How Long?_____

Water _____oz

Wake Time _____

Bed Time _____

How do I feel about today?

__ / __ / __

Food	Time	Hunger Level	Fullness Level	Emotion Before Eating	Emotion After Eating

Drink (non-water)

Exercise- YES   NO

Exercise Type_____

How Long?_____

Water _____oz

Wake Time _____

Bed Time _____

How do I feel about today?

___/___/___

Food	Time	Hunger Level	Fullness Level	Emotion Before Eating	Emotion After Eating

Drink (non-water)

Exercise- YES   NO

Exercise Type_____

How Long?_____

Water _____oz

Wake Time _____

Bed Time _____

How do I feel about today?

__ / __ / __

Food	Time	Hunger Level	Fullness Level	Emotion Before Eating	Emotion After Eating

Drink (non-water)

Exercise- YES   NO

Exercise Type_____

How Long?_____

Water _____oz

Wake Time _____

Bed Time _____

How do I feel about today?

__/__/__ Food	Time	Hunger Level	Fullness Level	Emotion Before Eating	Emotion After Eating

Drink (non-water)

Exercise- YES   NO

Exercise Type_____

How Long?_____

Water _____oz

Wake Time _____

Bed Time _____

How do I feel about today?

___/___/___

Food	Time	Hunger Level	Fullness Level	Emotion Before Eating	Emotion After Eating

Drink (non-water)

Exercise- YES   NO   Water _____oz
Exercise Type_____   Wake Time _____
How Long?_____   Bed Time _____

How do I feel about today?

___/___/___

Food	Time	Hunger Level	Fullness Level	Emotion Before Eating	Emotion After Eating

Drink (non-water)

	Time	Hunger Level	Fullness Level	Emotion Before Eating	Emotion After Eating

Exercise- YES   NO

Exercise Type_____

How Long?_____

Water _____oz

Wake Time _____

Bed Time _____

How do I feel about today?

___ / ___ / ___

Food	Time	Hunger Level	Fullness Level	Emotion Before Eating	Emotion After Eating

Drink (non-water)

Exercise- YES   NO

Exercise Type_____

How Long?_____

Water _____oz

Wake Time _____

Bed Time _____

How do I feel about today?

__/__/__ Food	Time	Hunger Level	Fullness Level	Emotion Before Eating	Emotion After Eating

Drink (non-water)

Exercise- YES   NO

Exercise Type_____

How Long?_____

Water _____oz

Wake Time _____

Bed Time _____

How do I feel about today?

_ / _ / _

Food	Time	Hunger Level	Fullness Level	Emotion Before Eating	Emotion After Eating

Drink (non-water)

Exercise- YES   NO   Water _____oz

Exercise Type_____   Wake Time _____

How Long?_____   Bed Time _____

How do I feel about today?

__/__/__

Food	Time	Hunger Level	Fullness Level	Emotion Before Eating	Emotion After Eating

Drink (non-water)

Exercise- YES   NO
Exercise Type_____
How Long?_____

Water _____oz
Wake Time _____
Bed Time _____

How do I feel about today?

___ / ___ / ___

Food	Time	Hunger Level	Fullness Level	Emotion Before Eating	Emotion After Eating

Drink (non-water)

Exercise- YES   NO

Exercise Type_____

How Long?_____

Water _____oz

Wake Time _____

Bed Time _____

How do I feel about today?

__ / __ / __

Food	Time	Hunger Level	Fullness Level	Emotion Before Eating	Emotion After Eating

Drink (non-water)

Exercise- YES   NO   Water _____ oz
Exercise Type _____   Wake Time _____
How Long? _____   Bed Time _____

How do I feel about today?

___/___/___

Food	Time	Hunger Level	Fullness Level	Emotion Before Eating	Emotion After Eating

Drink (non-water)

Exercise- YES   NO

Exercise Type_____

How Long?_____

Water _____oz

Wake Time _____

Bed Time _____

How do I feel about today?

___/___/___

Food	Time	Hunger Level	Fullness Level	Emotion Before Eating	Emotion After Eating

Drink (non-water)

Exercise- YES NO   Water _____oz

Exercise Type_____   Wake Time _____

How Long?_____   Bed Time _____

How do I feel about today?

___/___/___

Food	Time	Hunger Level	Fullness Level	Emotion Before Eating	Emotion After Eating

Drink (non-water)

	Time	Hunger Level	Fullness Level	Emotion Before Eating	Emotion After Eating

Exercise- YES   NO

Exercise Type_____

How Long?_____

Water _____oz

Wake Time _____

Bed Time _____

How do I feel about today?

___ / ___ / ___

Food

	Time	Hunger Level	Fullness Level	Emotion Before Eating	Emotion After Eating

Drink (non-water)

Exercise- YES   NO

Exercise Type_____

How Long?_____

Water _____ oz

Wake Time _____

Bed Time _____

How do I feel about today?

___/___/___

Food	Time	Hunger Level	Fullness Level	Emotion Before Eating	Emotion After Eating

Drink (non-water)

Exercise- YES   NO

Exercise Type_____

How Long?_____

Water _____oz

Wake Time _____

Bed Time _____

How do I feel about today?

___/___/___

Food	Time	Hunger Level	Fullness Level	Emotion Before Eating	Emotion After Eating

Drink (non-water)

	Time	Hunger Level	Fullness Level	Emotion Before Eating	Emotion After Eating

Exercise- YES   NO   Water _____oz
Exercise Type_____   Wake Time _____
How Long?_____   Bed Time _____

How do I feel about today?

____/____/____

Food	Time	Hunger Level	Fullness Level	Emotion Before Eating	Emotion After Eating

Drink (non-water)					

Exercise- YES   NO

Exercise Type_____

How Long?_____

Water _____ oz

Wake Time _____

Bed Time _____

How do I feel about today?

____/____/____

Food	Time	Hunger Level	Fullness Level	Emotion Before Eating	Emotion After Eating

Drink (non-water)

Exercise- YES   NO

Exercise Type_____

How Long?_____

Water _____oz

Wake Time _____

Bed Time _____

How do I feel about today?

___/___/___

Food	Time	Hunger Level	Fullness Level	Emotion Before Eating	Emotion After Eating

Drink (non-water)

	Time	Hunger Level	Fullness Level	Emotion Before Eating	Emotion After Eating

Exercise- YES   NO

Exercise Type_____

How Long?_____

Water _____oz

Wake Time _____

Bed Time _____

How do I feel about today?

__/__/__

Food	Time	Hunger Level	Fullness Level	Emotion Before Eating	Emotion After Eating

Drink (non-water)

	Time	Hunger Level	Fullness Level	Emotion Before Eating	Emotion After Eating

Exercise- YES   NO

Exercise Type_____

How Long?_____

Water _____oz

Wake Time _____

Bed Time _____

How do I feel about today?

___/___/___

Food	Time	Hunger Level	Fullness Level	Emotion Before Eating	Emotion After Eating

Drink (non-water)

Exercise- YES   NO

Exercise Type_____

How Long?_____

Water _____oz

Wake Time _____

Bed Time _____

How do I feel about today?

___/___/___

Food	Time	Hunger Level	Fullness Level	Emotion Before Eating	Emotion After Eating

Drink (non-water)

Exercise- YES   NO

Exercise Type_____

How Long?_____

Water _____ oz

Wake Time _____

Bed Time _____

How do I feel about today?

___/___/___

Food	Time	Hunger Level	Fullness Level	Emotion Before Eating	Emotion After Eating

Drink (non-water)

Exercise- YES   NO

Exercise Type_____

How Long?_____

Water _____oz

Wake Time _____

Bed Time _____

How do I feel about today?

___/___/___

Food	Time	Hunger Level	Fullness Level	Emotion Before Eating	Emotion After Eating

Drink (non-water)

Exercise- YES   NO   Water _____oz

Exercise Type_____   Wake Time _____

How Long?_____   Bed Time _____

How do I feel about today?

__/__/__

Food	Time	Hunger Level	Fullness Level	Emotion Before Eating	Emotion After Eating

Drink (non-water)

	Time	Hunger Level	Fullness Level	Emotion Before Eating	Emotion After Eating

Exercise- YES   NO

Exercise Type_____

How Long?_____

Water _____oz

Wake Time _____

Bed Time _____

How do I feel about today?

___/___/___

Food	Time	Hunger Level	Fullness Level	Emotion Before Eating	Emotion After Eating

Drink (non-water)

Exercise- YES   NO   Water _____oz
Exercise Type_____   Wake Time _____
How Long?_____   Bed Time _____

How do I feel about today?

___/___/___

Food	Time	Hunger Level	Fullness Level	Emotion Before Eating	Emotion After Eating

Drink (non-water)

	Time	Hunger Level	Fullness Level	Emotion Before Eating	Emotion After Eating

Exercise- YES   NO

Exercise Type_____

How Long?_____

Water _____oz

Wake Time _____

Bed Time _____

How do I feel about today?

___/___/___

Food	Time	Hunger Level	Fullness Level	Emotion Before Eating	Emotion After Eating

Drink (non-water)

	Time	Hunger Level	Fullness Level	Emotion Before Eating	Emotion After Eating

Exercise- YES   NO   Water _____oz
Exercise Type_____   Wake Time _____
How Long?_____   Bed Time _____

How do I feel about today?

__/__/__

Food	Time	Hunger Level	Fullness Level	Emotion Before Eating	Emotion After Eating

Drink (non-water)					

Exercise- YES   NO

Exercise Type_____

How Long?_____

Water _____oz

Wake Time _____

Bed Time _____

How do I feel about today?

___/___/___

Food	Time	Hunger Level	Fullness Level	Emotion Before Eating	Emotion After Eating

Drink (non-water)

Exercise- YES   NO

Exercise Type_____

How Long?_____

Water _____oz

Wake Time _____

Bed Time _____

How do I feel about today?

___ / ___ / ___

Food	Time	Hunger Level	Fullness Level	Emotion Before Eating	Emotion After Eating

Drink (non-water)					

Exercise- YES   NO

Exercise Type_____

How Long?_____

Water _____oz

Wake Time _____

Bed Time _____

How do I feel about today?

____/____/____

Food	Time	Hunger Level	Fullness Level	Emotion Before Eating	Emotion After Eating

Drink (non-water)

Exercise- YES   NO   Water _____oz
Exercise Type_____   Wake Time _____
How Long?_____   Bed Time _____

How do I feel about today?

___/___/___

Food	Time	Hunger Level	Fullness Level	Emotion Before Eating	Emotion After Eating

Drink (non-water)

Exercise- YES   NO

Exercise Type_____

How Long?_____

Water _____oz

Wake Time _____

Bed Time _____

How do I feel about today?

___/___/___

Food	Time	Hunger Level	Fullness Level	Emotion Before Eating	Emotion After Eating

Drink (non-water)

Exercise- YES   NO   Water _____oz
Exercise Type_____   Wake Time _____
How Long?_____   Bed Time _____

How do I feel about today?

___/___/___

Food	Time	Hunger Level	Fullness Level	Emotion Before Eating	Emotion After Eating

Drink (non-water)

Exercise- YES   NO

Exercise Type_____

How Long?_____

Water _____ oz

Wake Time _____

Bed Time _____

How do I feel about today?

_____ / _____ / _____

Food	Time	Hunger Level	Fullness Level	Emotion Before Eating	Emotion After Eating

Drink (non-water)

Exercise- YES   NO   Water _____oz
Exercise Type_____   Wake Time _____
How Long?_____   Bed Time _____

How do I feel about today?

___ / ___ / ___

Food	Time	Hunger Level	Fullness Level	Emotion Before Eating	Emotion After Eating

Drink (non-water)

	Time	Hunger Level	Fullness Level	Emotion Before Eating	Emotion After Eating

Exercise- YES   NO

Exercise Type_____

How Long?_____

Water _____oz

Wake Time _____

Bed Time _____

How do I feel about today?

_ _/_ _/_ _

Food	Time	Hunger Level	Fullness Level	Emotion Before Eating	Emotion After Eating

Drink (non-water)

Exercise- YES NO   Water _____oz

Exercise Type_____   Wake Time _____

How Long?_____   Bed Time _____

How do I feel about today?

__ / __ / __

Food	Time	Hunger Level	Fullness Level	Emotion Before Eating	Emotion After Eating

Drink (non-water)

Exercise- YES   NO

Exercise Type_____

How Long?_____

Water _____oz

Wake Time _____

Bed Time _____

How do I feel about today?

__ / __ / __

Food	Time	Hunger Level	Fullness Level	Emotion Before Eating	Emotion After Eating

Drink (non-water)

Exercise- YES   NO

Exercise Type_____

How Long?_____

Water _____oz

Wake Time _____

Bed Time _____

How do I feel about today?

___/___/___

Food

	Time	Hunger Level	Fullness Level	Emotion Before Eating	Emotion After Eating

Drink (non-water)

Exercise- YES   NO

Exercise Type_____

How Long?_____

Water _____oz

Wake Time _____

Bed Time _____

How do I feel about today?

____/____/____

Food	Time	Hunger Level	Fullness Level	Emotion Before Eating	Emotion After Eating

Drink (non-water)

	Time	Hunger Level	Fullness Level	Emotion Before Eating	Emotion After Eating

Exercise- YES   NO   Water _____ oz
Exercise Type_____   Wake Time _____
How Long?_____   Bed Time _____

How do I feel about today?

__/__/__ Food	Time	Hunger Level	Fullness Level	Emotion Before Eating	Emotion After Eating

Drink (non-water)					

Exercise- YES   NO

Exercise Type_____

How Long?_____

Water _____oz

Wake Time _____

Bed Time _____

How do I feel about today?

___/___/___

Food	Time	Hunger Level	Fullness Level	Emotion Before Eating	Emotion After Eating

Drink (non-water)

Exercise- YES   NO

Exercise Type_____

How Long?_____

Water _____oz

Wake Time _____

Bed Time _____

How do I feel about today?

___/___/___

Food	Time	Hunger Level	Fullness Level	Emotion Before Eating	Emotion After Eating

Drink (non-water)

Exercise- YES   NO

Exercise Type_____

How Long?_____

Water _____oz

Wake Time _____

Bed Time _____

How do I feel about today?

__/__/__

Food	Time	Hunger Level	Fullness Level	Emotion Before Eating	Emotion After Eating

Drink (non-water)

Exercise- YES   NO

Exercise Type_____

How Long?_____

Water _____oz

Wake Time _____

Bed Time _____

How do I feel about today?

___/___/___

Food	Time	Hunger Level	Fullness Level	Emotion Before Eating	Emotion After Eating

Drink (non-water)

Exercise- YES   NO

Exercise Type_____

How Long?_____

Water _____oz

Wake Time _____

Bed Time _____

How do I feel about today?

___/___/___

Food	Time	Hunger Level	Fullness Level	Emotion Before Eating	Emotion After Eating

Drink (non-water)

Exercise- YES   NO   Water _____oz
Exercise Type_____   Wake Time _____
How Long?_____   Bed Time _____

How do I feel about today?

___ / ___ / ___

Food	Time	Hunger Level	Fullness Level	Emotion Before Eating	Emotion After Eating

Drink (non-water)

Exercise- YES   NO

Exercise Type_____

How Long?_____

Water _____oz

Wake Time _____

Bed Time _____

How do I feel about today?

___/___/___

Food	Time	Hunger Level	Fullness Level	Emotion Before Eating	Emotion After Eating

Drink (non-water)					

Exercise- YES   NO

Exercise Type_____

How Long?_____

Water _____oz

Wake Time _____

Bed Time _____

How do I feel about today?

___/___/___

Food	Time	Hunger Level	Fullness Level	Emotion Before Eating	Emotion After Eating

Drink (non-water)

Exercise- YES   NO

Exercise Type_____

How Long?_____

Water _____oz

Wake Time _____

Bed Time _____

How do I feel about today?

___/___/___

Food	Time	Hunger Level	Fullness Level	Emotion Before Eating	Emotion After Eating

Drink (non-water)

	Time	Hunger Level	Fullness Level	Emotion Before Eating	Emotion After Eating

Exercise- YES   NO   Water _____oz
Exercise Type_____   Wake Time _____
How Long?_____   Bed Time _____

How do I feel about today?

___/___/___

Food	Time	Hunger Level	Fullness Level	Emotion Before Eating	Emotion After Eating

Drink (non-water)					

Exercise- YES   NO

Exercise Type_____

How Long?_____

Water _____oz

Wake Time _____

Bed Time _____

How do I feel about today?

___ / ___ / ___

Food	Time	Hunger Level	Fullness Level	Emotion Before Eating	Emotion After Eating

Drink (non-water)

Exercise- YES   NO   Water _____oz
Exercise Type_____   Wake Time _____
How Long?_____   Bed Time _____

How do I feel about today?

___/___/___

Food	Time	Hunger Level	Fullness Level	Emotion Before Eating	Emotion After Eating

Drink (non-water)

Exercise- YES   NO

Exercise Type_____

How Long?_____

Water _____oz

Wake Time _____

Bed Time _____

How do I feel about today?

___/___/___

Food	Time	Hunger Level	Fullness Level	Emotion Before Eating	Emotion After Eating

Drink (non-water)

	Time	Hunger Level	Fullness Level	Emotion Before Eating	Emotion After Eating

Exercise- YES   NO

Exercise Type_____

How Long?_____

Water _____oz

Wake Time _____

Bed Time _____

How do I feel about today?

___/___/___

Food	Time	Hunger Level	Fullness Level	Emotion Before Eating	Emotion After Eating

Drink (non-water)					

Exercise- YES   NO

Exercise Type_____

How Long?_____

Water _____oz

Wake Time _____

Bed Time _____

How do I feel about today?

___/___/___

Food	Time	Hunger Level	Fullness Level	Emotion Before Eating	Emotion After Eating

Drink (non-water)

Exercise- YES   NO

Exercise Type_____

How Long?_____

Water _____ oz

Wake Time _____

Bed Time _____

How do I feel about today?

___/___/___

Food

	Time	Hunger Level	Fullness Level	Emotion Before Eating	Emotion After Eating

Drink (non-water)

Exercise- YES   NO

Exercise Type_____

How Long?_____

Water _____oz

Wake Time _____

Bed Time _____

How do I feel about today?

__/__/__ Food	Time	Hunger Level	Fullness Level	Emotion Before Eating	Emotion After Eating

Drink (non-water)

Exercise- YES   NO

Exercise Type_____

How Long?_____

Water _____oz

Wake Time _____

Bed Time _____

How do I feel about today?

___/___/___

Food		Time	Hunger Level	Fullness Level	Emotion Before Eating	Emotion After Eating

Drink (non-water)

Exercise- YES   NO

Exercise Type_____

How Long?_____

Water _____oz

Wake Time _____

Bed Time _____

How do I feel about today?

____/____/____

Food

	Time	Hunger Level	Fullness Level	Emotion Before Eating	Emotion After Eating

Drink (non-water)

Exercise- YES   NO

Exercise Type_____

How Long?_____

Water _____oz

Wake Time _____

Bed Time _____

How do I feel about today?

___/___/___

Food	Time	Hunger Level	Fullness Level	Emotion Before Eating	Emotion After Eating

Drink (non-water)

	Time	Hunger Level	Fullness Level	Emotion Before Eating	Emotion After Eating

Exercise- YES   NO

Exercise Type_____

How Long?_____

Water _____oz

Wake Time _____

Bed Time _____

How do I feel about today?

___/___/___

Food	Time	Hunger Level	Fullness Level	Emotion Before Eating	Emotion After Eating

Drink (non-water)

Exercise- YES   NO   Water _____oz
Exercise Type_____   Wake Time _____
How Long?_____   Bed Time _____

How do I feel about today?

__ / __ / __

Food	Time	Hunger Level	Fullness Level	Emotion Before Eating	Emotion After Eating

Drink (non-water)

Exercise- YES   NO

Exercise Type_____

How Long?_____

Water _____oz

Wake Time _____

Bed Time _____

How do I feel about today?

___/___/___

Food	Time	Hunger Level	Fullness Level	Emotion Before Eating	Emotion After Eating

Drink (non-water)

Exercise- YES   NO

Exercise Type_____

How Long?_____

Water _____oz

Wake Time _____

Bed Time _____

How do I feel about today?

___/___/___

Food

	Time	Hunger Level	Fullness Level	Emotion Before Eating	Emotion After Eating

Drink (non-water)

Exercise- YES   NO

Exercise Type_____

How Long?_____

Water _____oz

Wake Time _____

Bed Time _____

How do I feel about today?

___/___/___

Food	Time	Hunger Level	Fullness Level	Emotion Before Eating	Emotion After Eating

Drink (non-water)

Exercise- YES   NO   Water _____ oz
Exercise Type_____   Wake Time _____
How Long?_____   Bed Time _____

How do I feel about today?

___/___/___

Food	Time	Hunger Level	Fullness Level	Emotion Before Eating	Emotion After Eating

Drink (non-water)

Exercise- YES   NO

Exercise Type_____

How Long?_____

Water _____oz

Wake Time _____

Bed Time _____

How do I feel about today?

___/___/___ Food	Time	Hunger Level	Fullness Level	Emotion Before Eating	Emotion After Eating

Drink (non-water)

Exercise- YES   NO

Exercise Type_____

How Long?_____

Water _____oz

Wake Time _____

Bed Time _____

How do I feel about today?

___ / ___ / ___

Food _____

	Time	Hunger Level	Fullness Level	Emotion Before Eating	Emotion After Eating

Drink (non-water)

Exercise- YES   NO

Exercise Type_____

How Long?_____

Water _____oz

Wake Time _____

Bed Time _____

How do I feel about today?

___ / ___ / ___

Food	Time	Hunger Level	Fullness Level	Emotion Before Eating	Emotion After Eating

Drink (non-water)

Exercise- YES   NO   Water _____ oz
Exercise Type_____   Wake Time _____
How Long?_____   Bed Time _____

How do I feel about today?

___/___/___

Food	Time	Hunger Level	Fullness Level	Emotion Before Eating	Emotion After Eating

Drink (non-water)

Exercise- YES   NO

Exercise Type_____

How Long?_____

Water _____oz

Wake Time _____

Bed Time _____

How do I feel about today?

__ / __ / __

Food	Time	Hunger Level	Fullness Level	Emotion Before Eating	Emotion After Eating

Drink (non-water)

Exercise- YES   NO

Exercise Type_____

How Long?_____

Water _____oz

Wake Time _____

Bed Time _____

How do I feel about today?

___ / ___ / ___

Food	Time	Hunger Level	Fullness Level	Emotion Before Eating	Emotion After Eating

Drink (non-water)					

Exercise- YES   NO

Exercise Type_____

How Long?_____

Water _____oz

Wake Time _____

Bed Time _____

How do I feel about today?

___/___/___

Food	Time	Hunger Level	Fullness Level	Emotion Before Eating	Emotion After Eating

Drink (non-water)

Exercise- YES   NO   Water _____oz
Exercise Type_____   Wake Time _____
How Long?_____   Bed Time _____

How do I feel about today?

_/_/_ Food	Time	Hunger Level	Fullness Level	Emotion Before Eating	Emotion After Eating

Drink (non-water)					

Exercise- YES   NO

Exercise Type_____

How Long?_____

Water _____oz

Wake Time _____

Bed Time _____

How do I feel about today?

___/___/___

Food	Time	Hunger Level	Fullness Level	Emotion Before Eating	Emotion After Eating

Drink (non-water)

	Time	Hunger Level	Fullness Level	Emotion Before Eating	Emotion After Eating

Exercise- YES   NO

Exercise Type_____

How Long?_____

Water _____oz

Wake Time _____

Bed Time _____

How do I feel about today?

___/___/___

Food	Time	Hunger Level	Fullness Level	Emotion Before Eating	Emotion After Eating

Drink (non-water)

	Time	Hunger Level	Fullness Level	Emotion Before Eating	Emotion After Eating

Exercise- YES   NO

Exercise Type_____

How Long?_____

Water _____oz

Wake Time _____

Bed Time _____

How do I feel about today?

___/___/___

Food	Time	Hunger Level	Fullness Level	Emotion Before Eating	Emotion After Eating

Drink (non-water)

Exercise- YES   NO   Water _____oz
Exercise Type_____   Wake Time _____
How Long?_____   Bed Time _____

How do I feel about today?

___/___/___

Food	Time	Hunger Level	Fullness Level	Emotion Before Eating	Emotion After Eating

Drink (non-water)

Exercise- YES   NO

Exercise Type_____

How Long?_____

Water _____oz

Wake Time _____

Bed Time _____

How do I feel about today?

__/__/__ Food	Time	Hunger Level	Fullness Level	Emotion Before Eating	Emotion After Eating

Drink (non-water)					

Exercise- YES   NO

Exercise Type_____

How Long?_____

Water _____oz

Wake Time _____

Bed Time _____

How do I feel about today?

___/___/___

Food	Time	Hunger Level	Fullness Level	Emotion Before Eating	Emotion After Eating

Drink (non-water)					

Exercise- YES   NO

Exercise Type_____

How Long?_____

Water _____oz

Wake Time _____

Bed Time _____

How do I feel about today?

___/___/___

Food	Time	Hunger Level	Fullness Level	Emotion Before Eating	Emotion After Eating

Drink (non-water)

Exercise- YES   NO

Exercise Type_____

How Long?_____

Water _____oz

Wake Time _____

Bed Time _____

How do I feel about today?

___/___/___

Food	Time	Hunger Level	Fullness Level	Emotion Before Eating	Emotion After Eating

Drink (non-water)

Exercise- YES   NO

Exercise Type_____

How Long?_____

Water _____oz

Wake Time _____

Bed Time _____

How do I feel about today?

____ / ____ / ____

Food	Time	Hunger Level	Fullness Level	Emotion Before Eating	Emotion After Eating

Drink (non-water)

Exercise- YES   NO

Exercise Type_____

How Long?_____

Water _____oz

Wake Time _____

Bed Time _____

How do I feel about today?

___/___/___

Food	Time	Hunger Level	Fullness Level	Emotion Before Eating	Emotion After Eating

Drink (non-water)

Exercise- YES   NO

Exercise Type_____

How Long?_____

Water _____oz

Wake Time _____

Bed Time _____

How do I feel about today?

_ _ / _ _ / _ _

Food	Time	Hunger Level	Fullness Level	Emotion Before Eating	Emotion After Eating

Drink (non-water)

Exercise- YES   NO   Water _____ oz
Exercise Type_____   Wake Time _____
How Long?_____   Bed Time _____

How do I feel about today?

___/___/___

Food

	Time	Hunger Level	Fullness Level	Emotion Before Eating	Emotion After Eating

Drink (non-water)

Exercise- YES   NO

Exercise Type_____

How Long?_____

Water _____oz

Wake Time _____

Bed Time _____

How do I feel about today?

___/___/___

Food	Time	Hunger Level	Fullness Level	Emotion Before Eating	Emotion After Eating

Drink (non-water)

Exercise- YES   NO

Exercise Type_____

How Long?_____

Water _____oz

Wake Time _____

Bed Time _____

How do I feel about today?

___/___/___

Food	Time	Hunger Level	Fullness Level	Emotion Before Eating	Emotion After Eating

Drink (non-water)

Exercise- YES   NO

Exercise Type_____

How Long?_____

Water _____oz

Wake Time _____

Bed Time _____

How do I feel about today?

___/___/___

Food	Time	Hunger Level	Fullness Level	Emotion Before Eating	Emotion After Eating

Drink (non-water)

Exercise- YES   NO

Exercise Type_____

How Long?_____

Water _____ oz

Wake Time _____

Bed Time _____

How do I feel about today?

_/__/__

Food	Time	Hunger Level	Fullness Level	Emotion Before Eating	Emotion After Eating

Drink (non-water)

Exercise- YES   NO

Exercise Type_____

How Long?_____

Water _____oz

Wake Time _____

Bed Time _____

How do I feel about today?

___/___/___

Food	Time	Hunger Level	Fullness Level	Emotion Before Eating	Emotion After Eating

Drink (non-water)

Exercise- YES   NO

Exercise Type_____

How Long?_____

Water _____oz

Wake Time _____

Bed Time _____

How do I feel about today?

___/___/___

Food	Time	Hunger Level	Fullness Level	Emotion Before Eating	Emotion After Eating

Drink (non-water)

Exercise- YES   NO

Exercise Type_____

How Long?_____

Water _____oz

Wake Time _____

Bed Time _____

How do I feel about today?

Notes

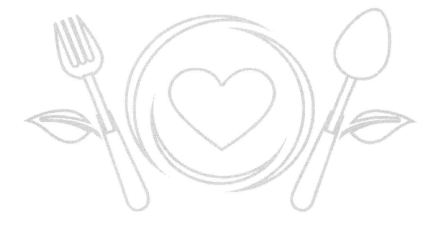

Notes

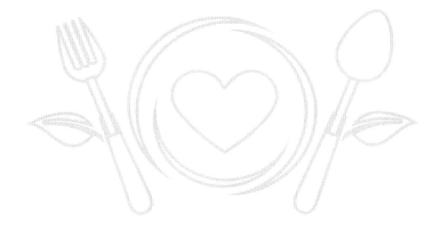

Notes

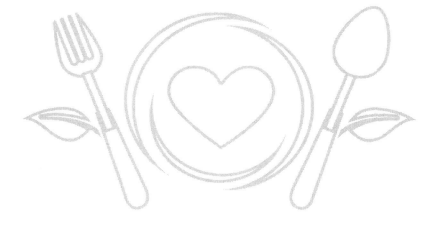

Notes

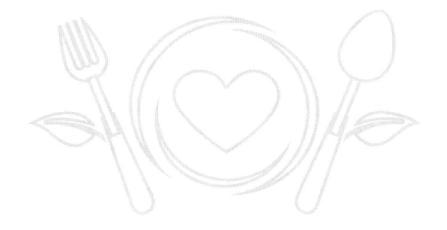

Notes

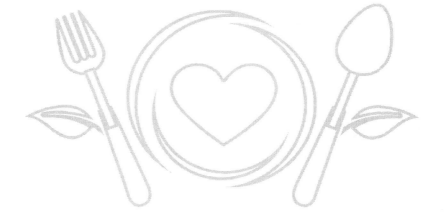

Notes

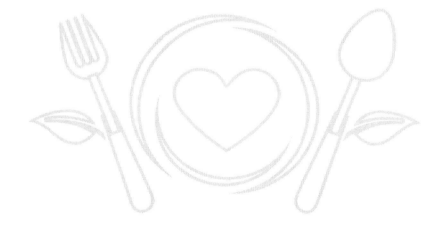

Notes

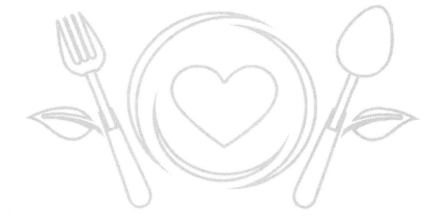

Notes

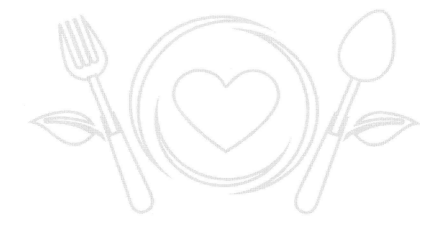

Notes

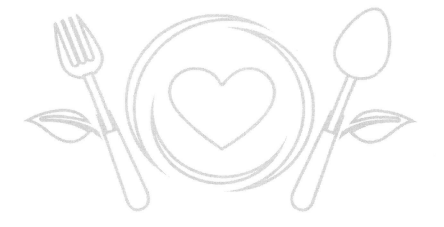

Notes

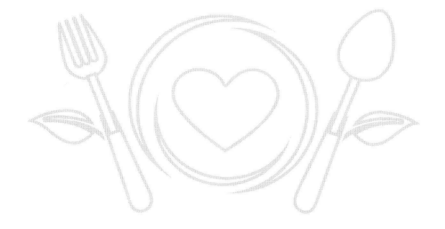

Notes

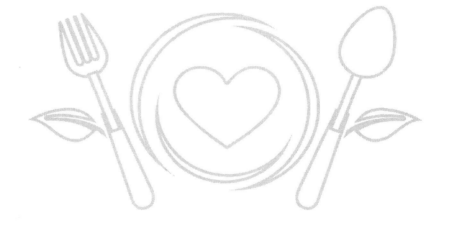

Notes

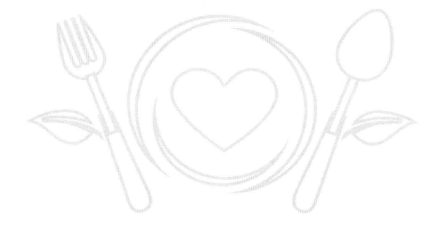

Notes

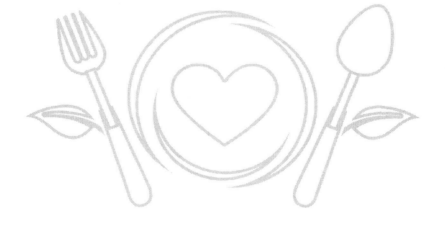

Notes

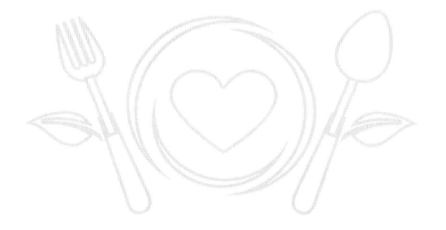

Notes

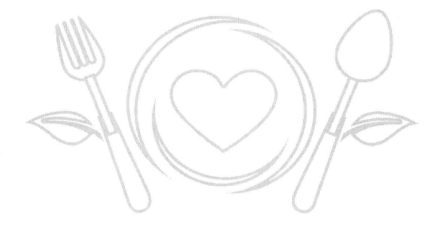

Made in the USA
Middletown, DE
08 October 2020

21441142R00113